Disclaimer and Safety Information

This information (and any accompanying material) is not intended to replace the attention or advice of a physician or other qualified health care professional. Anyone who wishes to embark on any dietary, drug, exercise, or other lifestyle change intended to prevent or treat a specific disease or condition should first consult with and seek clearance from a physician or other qualified health care professional. Pregnant women in particular should seek the advice of a physician before using any protocol listed in this book. The authors and publishers, their affiliates and assigns are not liable for any injury and/or damage to persons arising from this protocol and expressly disclaim responsibility for any adverse effects resulting from the use of the information contained herein.

Table of Contents

INTRODUCTION

Billions of people around the world are living with herpes infections, prompting the World Health Organization to call for a vaccine against the incurable virus. About half a billion people ages 15 to 49 have genital herpes infections, which are mostly caused by herpes simplex virus type 2, which can raise the risk of HIV. Herpes infections can lead to recurring, often painful, blisters. Genital herpes infections play a significant role in the spread of HIV globally according to report from World Health Organization.

Herpes is a very common skin disease. It's caused by a virus and can affect your mouth (oral) and/or the area around the penis or vagina (genital), upper thighs or buttocks. Most of the time, it is hard to notice herpes, so most people don't know they have it. Cold sores and fever blisters are an example of herpes in your mouth.

Anyone who has ever experienced shingles will know how frustrating a disease it can be. It is a viral condition which causes an incredibly painful rash, a rash which can crop up almost anywhere on the body. Most commonly, it appears as a strip of blisters that wraps around the torso on either side, but it can occur anywhere. If you have developed shingles, you are probably frustrated and maybe worried. Here we have for you natural ways to manage herpes and shingles of any kind you are battling to improve your immunity.

Forms of Herpes

Herpes simplex virus type 1 (HSV-1): this virus is contagious; its primary infection causes painful ulcers in the mouth in a child 1–3 years old. HSV-1 is capable of being dormant for months or years until cold sores appear. The attacks is triggered by emotional upset; fatigue and tiredness; colds or other viruses that weaken the body's defenses; menstrual periods; strong sunlight; cold winds.

Herpes genitalia (HSV-2): this infection is very similar to HSV-1 (50% of herpes genitalia are as a result of HSV-1); painful ulceration; dysuria; painful vaginal or urethral discharge; fever; myalgia; swollen lymph glands. It has more severe symptoms at initial attack than subsequently. It is also contagious.

Herpes zoster (shingles): Shingles, also known as herpes zoster or just zoster, occurs when a virus in nerve cells becomes active again later in life and causes a skin rash. The virus that causes shingles, the varicella-zoster virus, is the same virus that causes chickenpox. It is a member of the herpes virus family. Once you have had chickenpox, varicella-zoster virus remains in your body's nerve tissues and never really goes away. It is inactive, but it can be reactivated later in life. This causes shingles.

Symptom Progression:

- Starts with tingling sensation in affected area
- Fever and malaise may be present
- Erythema followed by blistering of the skin
- After five days, a one-sided rash appears, often over the ribs
- Blisters turn yellowish, flatten and dry out, and crust over
- Postherpetic neuralgia may occur following an attack due to nerve damage.

Differences Between Herpes and Shingles

There are many forms of Sexually Transmitted Infections/Diseases often abbreviated as (S.T.I'S/S.T.D'S). Some are common while others tend to be rare. Shingles and herpes are two common but varying types of such diseases. People tend to confuse the two; with others falsely asserting that shingles is a form of herpes. Shingles and herpes are two very different and distinct diseases.

They differ right from the onset based on their causative agents and continue to differ in their varied signs and symptoms, right up to their methods of transmission. Shingles is also referred to as herpes zoster in medical circles and herpes being referred to as herpes simplex. Due to the near similarity of their names, people tend to confuse them as being one and the same type of disease, which is to say the least far from the truth.

Shingles VS Herpes

The only similarity between these two diseases is the fact that they stem from the same family virus which is the herpes virus. There are eight known types of this virus. Herpes herein herpes simplex is caused by the Herpes Simplex Virus (H.S.V) which usually has two variants namely HSV-1 and HSV-2.

Shingles is caused by the Varicella Zoster Virus also known as HHV3 that also causes chicken pox. The difference does not end there. They also differ in their respective signs and symptoms and also in their varied modes of transmission and treatment.

Herpes

Herpes, also referred to as Herpes Simplex, is a contagious sexually transmitted disease that can be contracted during sexual intimacy. Its signs and symptoms are usually slow to appear and may take up to seven days prior to the first symptoms showing. In some people, they may take up to months and even years before showing. This is because this said virus may stay in one's body in a dormant state without necessarily leading to symptoms there and then. The duration prior to signs and symptoms appearing is hence dependent on a person's age and immune system.

Herpes Simplex: Signs and Symptoms

Many people who get the virus that causes herpes never see or feel anything. If signs (what you see) or symptoms (what you feel) occur, a person may experience:

- Tingling, itching, or burning. Before the blisters appear, the skin may tingle, itch, or burn for a day or so.
- Sores. One or more painful, fluid-filled blisters may appear. Blisters break open and often ooze fluid and form a crust, before healing. The first time sores appear, they will show up between 2 and 20 days after a person has contact with an infected person. The sores can last from 7 to 10 days. Where the sores appear often varies with type:
  - ✓ Oral herpes (HSV-1): Most blisters appear on the lips or around the mouth. Sometimes blisters form on the face or on

the tongue. Although these are the most common places to find oral herpes, the sores can appear anywhere on the skin.

- ✓ Genital herpes (HSV-2): Sores typically occur on the penis, vagina, buttocks, or anus. Women can have sores inside the vagina. Like oral herpes, these sores can appear anywhere on the skin.

- Flu-like symptoms. Fever, muscle aches, or swollen lymph nodes (glands) in the neck (oral herpes) or groin (genital herpes) are possible.

- Problems urinating. People (most often women) with genital herpes may have trouble urinating or have a burning feeling while urinating.

- An eye infection (herpes keratitis). Sometimes the herpes simplex virus can spread to one or both eyes. If this happens, you can have pain, light sensitivity, discharge, and a gritty feeling in the eye. Without prompt treatment, scarring of the eye may result. Scarring can lead to cloudy vision and even loss of vision.

If a person has HSV-1, bad sunburn can trigger a herpes simplex outbreak. If you develop signs and symptoms of herpes simplex, you can expect to have these for as long as listed below:

- Oral (mouth) herpes: two to three weeks
- Genital herpes: two to six weeks (the first outbreak)

Herpes simplex outbreaks usually develop around the mouth or on the genitals, but the sores can appear almost anywhere on the skin.

Diseases Caused by Herpes Simplex Virus

Diseases include

- Mucocutaneous infection (most common), including genital herpes
- Ocular infection (including herpes keratitis)
- Central nervous system (CNS) infection
- Neonatal herpes

HSV rarely causes fulminant hepatitis in the absence of cutaneous lesions.

In patients with HIV infection, herpetic infections can be particularly severe. Progressive and persistent esophagitis, colitis, perianal ulcers, pneumonia, encephalitis, and meningitis may occur.

HSV outbreaks may be followed by erythema multiforme, possibly caused by an immune reaction to the virus.

Eczema herpeticum is a complication of HSV infection in which severe herpetic disease develops in skin regions with eczema.

Mucocutaneous Herpes Simplex Infection

Lesions may appear anywhere on the skin or mucosa but are most frequent in the following locations:

- Mouth or lips (perioral infection)
- Genitals
- Conjunctiva and cornea

Generally, after a prodromal period (typically < 6 hours in recurrent HSV-1) of tingling discomfort or itching, clusters of small, tense vesicles appear on an erythematous base. Clusters vary in size from 0.5 to 1.5 cm but may coalesce. Lesions on the nose, ears, eyes, fingers, or genitals may be particularly painful.

Vesicles typically persist for a few days, then rupture and dry, forming a thin, yellowish crust.

Healing generally occurs within 10 to 19 days after onset in primary infection or within 5 to 10 days in recurrent infection. Lesions usually heal completely, but recurrent lesions at the same site may cause atrophy and scarring. Skin lesions can develop secondary bacterial infection. In patients with depressed cell-mediated immunity due to HIV infection or other conditions, prolonged or progressive lesions may persist for weeks or longer. Localized infections can disseminate, particularly and often dramatically in immunocompromised patients.

Acute Herpetic Gingivostomatitis usually results from primary infection with HSV-1, typically in children. Herpetic pharyngitis can occur in adults as well as children. Occasionally, through oral-genital contact, the cause is HSV-2. Intraoral and gingival vesicles rupture, usually within several hours to 1 or 2 days, to form ulcers. Fever and pain often occur. Difficulty eating and drinking may lead to dehydration. After resolution, the virus resides dormant in the semilunar ganglion.

Herpes Labialis is usually a recurrence of HSV. It develops as ulcers (cold sores) on the vermilion border of the lip or, much less commonly, as ulcerations of the mucosa of the hard palate.

Genital Herpes is the most common ulcerative sexually transmitted disease in developed countries. Genital HSV can be caused by HSV-1 or HSV-2.

Herpes Simplex Keratitis

Herpes simplex keratitis (HSV infection of the corneal epithelium) causes pain, tearing, photophobia, and corneal ulcers that often have a branching pattern.

Herpetic Whitlow

Herpetic whitlow, a swollen, painful, erythematous lesion of the finger, results from inoculation of HSV through the skin and is most common among health care practitioners.

Neonatal Herpes Simplex

Neonatal HSV infection develops in neonates, including those whose mothers have no suggestion of current or past herpes infection. It is most commonly transmitted during birth through contact with vaginal secretions containing HSV and usually involves HSV-2.

Neonatal HSV infection usually develops between the 1st and 4th week of life, often causing mucocutaneous vesicles or central nervous system involvement. It causes major morbidity and mortality.

Herpes Simplex CNS Infection

Herpes encephalitis occurs sporadically and may be severe. Multiple early seizures are characteristic.

Viral Meningitis may result from HSV-2. It is usually self-limited.

Lumbosacral myeloradiculitis, typically caused by HSV-2, can occur during primary infection and can result in urinary retention or obstipation.

Who Can be infected by Herpes Simplex?

Most people get HSV-1 (herpes simplex type 1) as an infant or child. This virus can be spread by skin-to-skin contact with an adult who carries the virus. An adult does not have to have sores to spread the virus.

A person usually gets HSV-2 (herpes simplex type 2) through sexual contact. About 20% of sexually active adults in the United States carry HSV-2. Some people are more likely to get HSV-2. These people:

- Are female
- Have had many sex partners
- Had sex for the first time at a young age
- Have (or had) another sexually transmitted infection
- Have a weakened immune system due to a disease or medicine

Root Cause of Herpes Simplex

Herpes simplex viruses spread from person to person through close contact. You can get a herpes simplex virus from touching a herpes sore. Most people, however, get herpes simplex from an infected person who does not have sores. Doctors call this "asymptomatic viral shedding."

How people get herpes around their mouth

A person with HSV-1 (herpes simplex type 1) can pass it to someone else by:

- Kissing
- Touching the person's skin, such as pinching a child's cheek
- Sharing objects such as silverware, lip balm, or a razor

How people get herpes on their genitals

You can get genital herpes after coming into contact with HSV-1 or HSV-2. Most people get genital herpes from HSV-2, which they get during sex. If someone has a cold sore and performs oral sex, this can spread HSV-1 to the genitals, and cause herpes sores on the genitals.

Mothers can give the herpes virus to their baby during childbirth. If the baby is born during the mother's first episode of genital herpes, the baby can have serious problems.

What happens once you have HSV-1 or HSV-2?

Once a person becomes infected with a herpes virus, the virus never leaves the body. After the first outbreak, the virus moves from the skin cells to nerve cells. The virus stays in the nerve cells forever. But it usually just stays there. In this stage, the virus is said to be dormant, or asleep. But it can become active again.

Some things that can trigger (wake up) the virus are:

- Stress
- Illness
- Fever
- Sun exposure
- Menstrual periods
- Surgery

Shingles

Also referred to as Herpes Zoster, is a type of the Herpes Human Virus, caused by the Varicella Zoster virus (HHV-3) that is also responsible for causing chickenpox. Shingles is different from herpes as they are caused by different types of the Herpes Human Virus. This virus is chronic, so, despite treatment, the virus still remains in one's body and may be triggered to recur again after sometime. For Shingles in particular, the virus tends to stay in one's nerve tissue, which is located near one's spinal cord and brain until when it is triggered. Upon being triggered, it travels down to the closest skin tissue and manifests itself as a rash, usually on the neck or torso. It tends to be more prevalent in older adults and persons with weak immune systems. Shingles, unlike Herpes, is not contagious. It cannot be passed on, however, there is a small chance that it can be passed on to someone who has not gotten chicken pox or its vaccine. Should it be passed on to such a person, they may suffer from shingles later in life.

Symptoms of Shingles

Symptoms occur in the area of skin that is supplied by the affected nerve fibres. The usual symptoms are pain and a rash. Occasionally, two or three nerves next to each other are affected. Very rarely, shingles can affect both sides of the body, but this is usually in people with a weakened immune system.

The most commonly involved nerves are those supplying the skin on the chest or tummy (abdomen). The upper face (including an eye) is also a common site.

The pain is a localised band of pain. It can be anywhere on your body, depending on which nerve is affected. The pain can range from mild to severe. You may have a constant dull, burning, or gnawing pain. In addition, or instead, you may have sharp and stabbing pains that come and go. The affected area of skin is usually tender.

The rash typically appears 2-3 days after the pain begins. Red blotches appear that quickly develop into itchy fluid-filled blisters. The rash looks like chickenpox but only appears on the band of skin supplied by the affected nerve. New blisters may appear for up to a week. The soft tissues under and around the rash may become swollen for a while due to inflammation caused by the virus. The blisters then dry up, form scabs and gradually fade away. Slight scarring may occur where the blisters have been. The picture shows a scabbing rash (a few days old) of a fairly bad bout of shingles. In this person, it has affected a nerve and the skin that the nerve supplies, on the left side of the abdomen.

Signs of Shingles

An episode of shingles usually lasts 2-4 weeks. In some cases there is a rash but no pain. Rarely, there is no rash but just a band of pain.

You may also feel you have a high temperature (feel feverish) and feel unwell for a few days.

Is shingles contagious?

You can catch chickenpox from someone with shingles if you have not had chickenpox before. But most adults and older children have already had chickenpox and so are immune from catching chickenpox again. You cannot get shingles from someone who has shingles.

The shingles rash is contagious (for someone else to catch chickenpox) until all the blisters (vesicles) have scabbed and are dry. If the blisters are covered with a dressing, it is unlikely that the virus will pass on to others. This is because the virus is passed on by direct contact with the blisters. If you have a job, you can return to work once the blisters have dried up, or earlier if you keep the rash covered and feel well enough. Similarly children with shingles can go to school if the rash is covered by clothes and they do not feel unwell.

Pregnant women who have not had chickenpox should avoid people with shingles.

Also, if you have a poor immune system (immunosuppression), you should avoid people with shingles. (See below for a list of people who have a poor immune system.) These general rules are to be on the safe side, as it is direct contact with the rash that usually passes on the virus.

Can other people catch it?

This one is confusing! You can catch chickenpox from other people, but you can't catch shingles from other people. You only get shingles from a reactivation of your own chickenpox infection in the past.

So if you have shingles, and you come into contact with somebody else, they cannot 'catch' your shingles. But if they have never had chickenpox, it is possible that they could catch chickenpox from you. (And if you had chickenpox, and came into contact with somebody else who had never had chickenpox, they could catch chickenpox. But they couldn't 'catch' shingles from your chickenpox.)

To put it another way, no, you don't 'catch' shingles. It comes from a virus hiding out in your own body, not from someone else. But if you have shingles, you may be infectious, as it is possible for people to catch chickenpox from you.

Only people who have never had chickenpox are likely to be at risk of catching chickenpox from your shingles. People who have had chickenpox should be immune from catching it again. If the rash is in a covered area of skin, the risk of anyone with whom you are not in close contact catching chickenpox is very low.

How common is it?

Shingles is an infection of a nerve and the area of skin supplied by the nerve. It is caused by a virus called the varicella-zoster virus. It is the same virus that causes chickenpox. Anyone who has had chickenpox in the past may develop shingles. Shingles is sometimes called herpes zoster. (Note: this is very different to genital herpes which is caused by a different virus called herpes simplex.)

About 1 in 4 people have shingles at some time in their lives. It can occur at any age but it is most common in older adults (over the age of 50 years). After the age of 50, it becomes increasingly more common as you get older. It is uncommon to have shingles more than once but some people do have it more than once.

Causes of Shingles

Most people have chickenpox at some stage (usually as a child). The virus does not completely go after you have chickenpox. Some virus particles remain inactive in the nerve roots next to your spinal cord. They do no harm there and cause no symptoms. For reasons that are not clear, the virus may begin to multiply again (reactivate). This is often years later. The reactivated virus travels along the nerve to the skin to cause shingles.

In most cases, an episode of shingles occurs for no apparent reason. Sometimes a period of stress or illness seems to trigger it. A slight ageing of the immune system may account for it being more common in older people. (The immune system keeps the virus inactive and prevents it from multiplying. A slight weakening of the immune system in older people may account for the virus reactivating and multiplying to cause shingles.)

The risk of getting shingles increases in people with a poor immune system (immunosuppression). For example, shingles commonly occurs in younger people who have HIV/AIDS or whose immune system is suppressed with treatment such as steroids or chemotherapy.

When It Feels Like Shingles but It's Really Something Else

Even if you've heard of shingles and know that it's a painful rash, you still might have a hard time knowing for sure if it is the cause of your symptoms.

Shingles has two features that distinguish it from conditions with similar symptoms: its flu-like onset and the severe pain that follows.

The list below is no substitute for a doctor's diagnosis, but the following descriptions of other skin reactions may help you determine what you don't have before you call your doctor, which you should absolutely do if these symptoms appear.

Here's how other skin reactions manifest on the skin:

- The Herpes Simplex Virus Symptoms are usually seen around the mouth or genitals.
- An Allergic Reaction on the Skin An allergic reaction isn't bumpy, but usually appears red, swollen, and irregular in shape.
- Hives These are red, itchy, and swollen bumps that can appear anywhere on the body.
- Eczema Like shingles, eczema can consist of oozing blisters, but it's primarily scaly and flaky.
- Psoriasis This condition is also scaly and flaky.
- Bed Bug Bites These are also red and bumpy patches that itch, but they will likely show up

on your arms or legs, and can often appear in a straight line.

Treatment of Herpes

There are several known ways of treating herpes. They are outlined below:

1. Uptake of Vitamin C and Zinc which helps and greatly facilitates in boosting one's natural immunity so as to combat the said disease then and in future, should it reoccur.

2. Paracetamols may be prescribed so as to ease the pain caused by the symptoms, in some cases the pain may be dire.

3. Persons with the said infection have reported feeling a temporary relief once they take a warm bath, sometimes laced with a little bit of salt.

4. Strong anti-viral drugs may be prescribed to combat the said virus, such as acyclovir, however, they do not serve to cure the virus as it is chronic.

5. One may use Vaseline or any other viable petroleum jelly or aloe vera to apply on the affected areas with blisters. This aids in soothing them and hastening their healing process. It also prevents their rupture, which would consequently lead to unwanted secondary infections in the affected area. Hygiene is also a key to the problem, while dealing with the respective blisters to avoid their contamination.

Treatment of Shingles

There are various modes of treating herpes zoster or shingles. However, the fact that it is caused by a virus means it cannot be removed from one's body completely. It is a chronic illness and may thus recur from time to time even after treatment, depending on one's age and natural immunity level.

Age and immunity level are the determinants on recurrence. The various methods of treatment are as listed below:

1. The use of anti-viral drugs such as acyclovir, or famciclovir under the brand name Famvir may be prescribed to a patient.

2. Painkillers or pain relievers may be prescribed when the pain is excessive and excruciating by medical standards. In dire cases, narcotic consisting medication may be given, such as opoids which include codeine.

3. There are available vaccines in most medical hospitals and approved clinics which assist in curbing of this infection.

4. In some instances, under the discretion of a certified medical practitioner, paracetamols may be prescribed, so as to reduce the pain emanating from this infection.

5. As the rashes tend to rupture, sometimes becoming susceptible to secondary infections, one is advised to use Calamine lotion as it helps curb secondary infections, keeping them at bay.

Best Home Remedies For Herpes

Thankfully, there are several effective home remedies for herpes

1. Ice Pack

Procedure:

- Take a handful of ice cubes. Wrap them up in a plastic bag.
- Apply gently on the blisters.
- Repeat the cold compress 2 to 3 times daily for a week.

How does this work?

An ice pack is a universal remedy for wounds and blisters as it helps control the swelling and gives relief from the pain. The ice pack works on the underlying tissue and offers relief from the pain and burning sensation caused by the blisters caused by Herpes.

Repeated application of cold compresses helps keep the blisters from accumulating fluid and bursting. Ice pack remedies are easy to administer, making them one of the favorite home remedies for Herpes outbreaks.

Additionally, water also plays an important role here. With water getting impure day by day, it is causing severe effects on our health and day-to-day activities. Make sure you drink purified water such as a technique called reverse osmosis system to ensure healthy water.

The Remedy is not Good if:

The ice cubes are applied directly on the blisters as the water can enter inside the wound and cause infection.

2. Baking Soda

Procedure:

- Mix 2 to 3 teaspoons of baking soda (sodium bicarbonate) in a glass of warm water.
- Take a few balls of surgical cotton. Dip it in the solution and apply on the blisters.
- Repeat the process 2 to 3 times in the course of the day.

How does this work?

Baking soda has been praised as one of the best home remedies and has many applications. It has a mild alkaline effect and has a soothing effect on the blisters. Baking soda offers relief from the burning and itching sensation caused by Herpes blisters and eases the pain as well.

It is a great anti-inflammatory agent and helps reduce the swelling caused by blistering wounds. The ease with which baking soda can be used to treat Herpes makes it one of the favorite home remedies for Herpes outbreaks.

The Remedy is not Good if:

There is no reason why baking soda won't work on blisters caused by Herpes. Moreover, it has no side effects, making it safe to use.

3. Tea Tree Oil

Procedure:

- Add 2 to 3 teaspoons of undiluted tea tree oil in a glass of warm water.
- Take a few balls of surgical cotton. Dip it in the solution and apply on the blisters.
- Gargle the mouth if ulcers are present in the mouth.
- Repeat the process twice daily for a week.

How does this work?

The benefits of tea tree oil have been extolled in various texts and the aborigines of Australia have used it for centuries for its curative properties. Tea tree oil is used as an additive in many skin and hair care products like deodorants, disinfectants, soap oils, soaps, and face and body lotions. The soothing effect this oil has on the blisters caused by Herpes gives instant relief from the pain and burning.

However, care should be taken to ensure that none of the oil gets into the eyes as it can cause irritation and redness. However, the therapeutic effects of tea tree oil make it one of the best home remedies for herpes outbreak.

The Remedy is not Good if:

The tea tree oil enters the eyes as it can cause severe irritation and redness. Otherwise, there are no side effects attributed to tea tree oil.

4. Licorice Powder

Procedure:

- Mix 2 teaspoons of licorice root powder in some water to make a paste.
- Apply the paste gently on the blisters.
- Let it sit for an hour or so. Repeat the process twice daily for a week.

How does this work?

Licorice root helps build up a strong immune system and helps in fighting the Herpes outbreak in a patient. Licorice also has strong anti-viral and anti-bacterial properties, thanks to the ingredient glycyrthizin found in it in abundant quantities.

Licorice powder can be mixed in warm water and consumed internally as well as it enhances the immune system. However, people with a history of hypertension should refrain from consuming it as it can trigger the blood pressure. However, there is no denying the fact that licorice is one of the best remedies for herpes outbreaks.

The Remedy is not Good if:

You are a hypertension patient (high blood pressure) as it can trigger your blood pressure and cause it to rise.

5. Garlic in Olive Oil

Procedure:

- Take 2 to 3 pods of garlic, wash, and peel. Crush the garlic pods.
- Take 100 ml of virgin olive oil. Heat the olive oil in a bowl and add the garlic.
- Allow simmering for 5 minutes. Strain the oil and apply on the blisters.
- Repeat the process twice daily for a week.

How does this work?

Garlic is another wonder herb that is loaded with beneficial properties. The benefits of the herb have been extolled in various texts and it has been used as medicine for hundreds of years. It has high anti-microbial properties as well as anti-inflammatory properties that help heal the blisters caused by Herpes and helps in containing the swelling.

Garlic also has anti-viral properties due to the presence of the compounds allicin and ajoene. As raw garlic can be harsh on the raw blisters and wounds, it is treated with olive oil to reduce the harshness yet retain the curative effects.

The Remedy is not Good if:

There is no reason why this remedy won't be good in treating Herpes outbreaks.

6. Aloe Vera and Turmeric

Procedure:

- Cut a thick leaf of Aloe Vera. Remove the thorny edges on either side.
- Peel the skin on the rounded side and collect the gel.
- Take 2 teaspoons of organic Turmeric and mix with Aloe Vera gel.
- Apply the paste on the blisters and allow to sit for an hour.
- Repeat the process twice daily for a week.

How does this work?

Aloe Vera is the hardy wonder herb that has multiple medicinal applications. Apart from being consumed internally for various disorders, it is a great skin restorer and acts as a natural antiseptic agent. Aloe Vera also has excellent anti-microbial properties and helps cure the infection incredibly fast.

Turmeric is a magic spice that has curative powers that are extolled in various Ayurvedic texts. It is a natural antiseptic and helps heal severe wounds, and helps in curing the blisters caused by Herpes. This wonderful combination is probably the safest and most effective of all home remedies for Herpes.

The Remedy is not Good if:

There is no way this remedy cannot be good. It has no side effects and is a strong cure for Herpes.

7. Lemon Balm

Procedure:

- Mix 2 to 3 teaspoons of lemon balm tincture (Amazon) in a glass of warm water.
- Take a few balls of surgical cotton.

- Dip it in the solution and apply on the blisters or sores.
- Repeat the process a couple of times a day for a week.

How does this work?

Lemon balm tincture is very effective in controlling Herpes and offers instant relief from the pain and itching. This tincture is loaded with flavonoids that work wonders for Herpes infection. Moreover, the phenolic acid and rosmarinic acid content in Lemon balm tincture have a soothing effect on the burning wounds and act as salves.

Apart from applying locally, lemon balm tea can be prepared and consumed. Even adding a few drops of the tincture in water and drinking it regularly for a week gives relief from Herpes. All these qualities make Lemon balm tincture one of the most popular home remedies for Herpes outbreaks.

The Remedy is not Good if:

The infection is severe and requires immediate medical attention.

Treatment is given long after the Herpes infection sets in.

8. Hydrogen Peroxide

Procedure:

- Take 2 to 3 teaspoons of Hydrogen Peroxide of 3% proof.
- Take a few balls of surgical cotton.
- Dip in the Hydrogen Peroxide and apply gently.
- For sores in the mouth, dilute Hydrogen Peroxide with 4 parts water.
- Repeat the process 2 to 3 times a week for two weeks.

How does this work?

Hydrogen Peroxide is an excellent disinfectant and helps clean the blisters and wounds caused by Herpes. It also has a curative effect and helps control the itching and burning sensation associated with Herpes.

It is also an excellent anti-microbial agent and helps contain the infection and hastens the healing process. If the wounds are too severe, it is better to dilute the Hydrogen Peroxide as 3% proof may be too harsh on raw wounds. Hydrogen Peroxide is one of the best home remedies for Herpes outbreak and helps contain it successfully.

The Remedy is not Good if:

The wounds are raw and too severe. This can cause a burning sensation and aggravate the pain.

Used as a mouthwash without diluting the 3% Hydrogen Peroxide as it can cause a severe burning sensation in the ulcers in the mouth.

9. Tea Bags

Procedure:

- Boil 2 to 3 tea bags in a glass of water.
- Take a few balls of surgical cotton. Dip in lukewarm tea decoction.
- Apply on the affected parts. Repeat the process twice daily for a week.

How does this work?

Black tea contains rich quantities of tannin. The tannin content in the tea gives it strong anti-viral properties that help control the Herpes virus. Moreover, tea also contains anti-inflammatory properties that help in keeping the swelling under control. Apply the tea decoction on the blisters and raw wounds help hasten the speeding process and also gives immense relief from the pain as well as the itching and burning sensation. Moreover, this remedy is so easy to make which is probably why it is one of the most sought after home remedies for herpes.

The Remedy is not Good if:

It is a severe case of infection with other symptoms like persistent fever.

There is no sign of any improvement and the blisters ulcers do not subside.

10. Apple Cider Vinegar

Procedure:

- Take 2 to 3 teaspoons of undiluted apple cider vinegar (ACV).
- Take a few balls of surgical cotton.
- Dip the cotton balls in ACV and apply on affected portions.

- If the infection is very severe, dilute the ACV before using.
- Repeat the process twice daily for a week or so.

How does this work?

Apple cider vinegar has great disinfectant properties and is also a strong astringent that helps repair the body tissues and canals. ACV also has high anti-inflammatory properties that help reduce the swelling caused by the Herpes virus. Applying ACV on the affected parts has a soothing effect and gives great relief from the itching and burning sensation associated with Herpes.

Take care not to apply undiluted ACV on raw wounds that are severe in nature as it can cause a severe burning sensation. In such cases, it is better to dilute the ACV before using. Whichever form apple cider vinegar is used, it is one of the best home remedies for herpes outbreaks.

The Remedy is not Good if:

The infection is too severe as applying undiluted apple cider vinegar can cause an intense burning sensation and have contra effects.

Topical Herbs, Oils, and Other Solutions

11. Echinacea

Echinacea is a medicinal plant and has anti-viral properties. It is known for enhancing the immune system and easing the symptoms of this viral infection. All parts of the Echinacea plant, namely flowers, leaves, and roots can be used for healing herpes.

What to do:

• You can consume echinacea as tea, juices, or pills. Depending on the form you want, try getting the recommended dose every day.

12. Cornstarch

One of the best home remedies for herpes is cornstarch. Cornstarch helps in absorbing excessive moisture from the skin. It helps in reducing chafing and itching.

What to do:

- Apply some cornstarch directly on the infected area.
- Take a cotton ball and dip it in the cornstarch.
- Dab it gently on the sores.
- To circumvent contamination, do not put used cotton ball again in the clean cornstarch.

13. Epsom Salt

Another home remedy for herpes is bathing in Epsom salt water. It is a perfect remedy for soothing the itching and pain in herpes. This remedy makes the sores dry, thereby reducing itching.

What to do:

- Add some Epsom salt in warm bathing water.
- Take a bath from it.
- You can also add some salt in the bathtub.
- Soak herpes infected area in the water.
- Allow it to dry and then, take a shower.

14. Domeboro Powder

Domeboro powder can be used for healing the herpes infection. It can be used on the sores in the form of a compressor as wet dressing. The powder helps in soothing the irritated and itchy skin.

What to do:

- Mix one packet of domeboro powder in water as per the directions on the packet.
- Now, dip a piece of clean cloth in the solution.
- Apply the cloth directly on the infected area.

15. Lysine

One of the other natural remedies for herpes is lysine. It is a kind of amino acids that are found in foods, including milk, brewer's yeast, cheeses, chicken, etc. It is known for reducing herpes outbreak.

What to do:

- Look for lysine cream on the market.
- Apply it to the infected areas according to the indications.

16. Black Coffee

Herpes virus infects not only genital parts but also lips, mouth, etc. Black coffee is one of the best remedies to treat them. Blisters in the mouth cause severe pain.

What to do:

- Prepare black coffee.
- Let it cool down and take a sip.
- Hold it in the mouth for some time.
- Move it to the lips as well.
- For best results, repeat the process twice a day.

17. Soap and Warm Water

Surprisingly, warm water can have an unexpected effect on plenty of health issues. For example, soaking the herpes sore in warm water surely relieves the pain and itching.

What to do:

- Soak the affected area in warm water.
- Add soap to keep the area infection-free and clean.
- Don't forget to dry your genital parts with a clean towel.
- Do not share a bathtub with an infected person.

18. Herbal Tea

Herbal tea is an effective solution for avoiding any type of skin diseases. For treating pain and itching arising due to herpes, herbal teas, like lemon, ginger, cinnamon, and chamomile are very effective.

What to do:

- Choose your favorite plant from the list above.
- Let it infuse and drink the tea a couple of times a day.

- Combine different plants according to your preferences.

19. Manuka Honey

Manuka honey has antibacterial and anti-viral properties. It helps in quick healing of herpes blisters. Moreover, it's one of the best home remedies for cold sores.

What to do:

- Apply some manuka honey directly on the infected area.

20. Over-the-counter Medicines

Pain relievers or over-the-counter analgesics are useful in relieving the aching herpes outburst.

What to do:

- Use some of the OTC medications that include ibuprofen, acetaminophen, and aspirin.
- To treat herpes sores, some ointments, like propolis, can also be applied to the infected area.

21. Natural Oils

Natural oils are effective in relieving the herpes ache and itching. Olive, jojoba, tea tree, vitamin E, camellia, and calendula oils are known for fighting against the virus.

What to do:

- Apply any of the natural oil or mixture of some oils on the infected area, gently. This will heal the infected skin.

22. Goldenseal

Goldenseal is another natural herpes treatment. It's a good solution if you want to get rid of this problem at home quickly.

What to do:

- Take some walnut hull powder and add Echinacea and goldenseal in it.
- Stir it well to make a paste.
- Apply the paste to the infected area.
- Goldenseal is also available in pills, tincture, salve, and bulk powder.

23. Oregano Oil

Oregano oil, with its anti-viral properties, can help alleviate the symptoms of the herpes simplex virus and helps in the speedy recovery of herpes blisters. You can also use coconut oil as another herpes treatment alongside oregano oil.

What to do:

- You just need to apply some oregano oil directly on the infected area.

24. Witch Hazel

Witch hazel has significant antiviral properties. Some people can use pure witch hazel without experiencing irritation, while others find that it stings. You should use a diluted solution if you have sensitive skin.

25. Goat Milk

Goat milk contains an antiviral agent that may work against herpes simplex. You can apply goat milk directly without dilution.

26. Chamomile Essential Oil

Some research suggests that chamomile essential oil has soothing and virus-fighting properties that may help treat HSV-2. It must be diluted with a carrier oil.

27. Thyme Essential Oil

Thyme essential oil also has potential to fight the herpes virus. It must be diluted with a carrier oil.

28. Greek Sage Oil

Greek sage oil may also fight the herpes virus. It must be diluted with a carrier oil.

29. Eucalyptus Oil

Eucalyptus oil may be a potent antiviral against herpes. It also soothes and promotes healing. It must be diluted with a carrier oil.

30. Mexican Oregano Oil

Mexican oregano oil contains carvacrol, a powerful antiviral ingredient. It must be diluted with a carrier oil.

31. Neem Extract

Neem extract may also have significant anti-herpes properties. Pure Neem extract is potent and may burn your skin. It must be diluted with a carrier oil.

General do's and don'ts

Here are some general tips for outbreak management.

If you have a cold sore.

- DO ditch your toothbrush and use a new one.
- DO load up on rest, vitamin C, and zinc supplements when you're experiencing high stress.
- DO use a hypoallergenic, clear lip balm to protect your skin from sun, wind, and cold exposure.
- DON'T share cups or drinks during the outbreak.

- DON'T try to pop, drain, or otherwise interfere with the cold sore while it's healing.

If you have a genital herpes outbreak...

- DO wear cotton undergarments and loose clothing.
- DO take long warm showers and keep the area clean and dry at all other times.
- DON'T soak in hot tubs or baths.
- DON'T have sex. It's possible to transmit the virus even if you use a condom.

Painkillers for Shingles

Painkillers - for example, paracetamol, or paracetamol combined with codeine (such as co-codamol), or anti-inflammatory painkillers (such as ibuprofen) - may give some relief. Strong painkillers (such as oxycodone and tramadol) may be needed in some cases.

Some painkillers are particularly useful for nerve pain. If the pain during an episode of shingles is severe, or if you develop postherpetic neuralgia (PHN), you may be advised to take:

- An antidepressant medicine in the tricyclic group. An antidepressant is not used here to treat depression. Tricyclic antidepressants, such as amitriptyline, imipramine and nortriptyline, ease nerve pain (neuralgia) separate to their action on depression; or
- An anticonvulsant medicine such as gabapentin or pregabalin. They also ease neuralgic pain separate to their action to control convulsions.

If an antidepressant or anticonvulsant is advised, you should take it regularly as prescribed. It may take up to two or more weeks for it to become fully effective to ease pain. In addition to easing pain during an episode of shingles, they may also help to prevent PHN.

Antiviral Medicines for Shingles

Antiviral medicines used to treat shingles include aciclovir, famciclovir and valaciclovir. An antiviral medicine does not kill the virus but works by stopping the virus from multiplying. So, it may limit the severity of symptoms of the shingles episode.

An antiviral medicine is most useful when started in the early stages of shingles (within 72 hours of the rash appearing). However, in some cases your doctor may still advise you have an antiviral medicine even if the rash is more than 72 hours old particularly in elderly people with severe shingles, or if shingles affects an eye.

Antiviral medicines are not advised routinely for everybody with shingles. As a general rule, the following groups of people who develop shingles will normally be advised to take an antiviral medicine:

• If you are over the age of 50. The older you are, the more risk there is of severe shingles or complications developing and the more likely you are to benefit from treatment.

• If you are of any age and have any of the following:

> Shingles that affects the eye or ear.
> A poorly functioning immune system (immunosuppression - see later for who is included).
> Shingles that affects any parts of the body apart from the trunk (that is, shingles affecting an arm, leg, neck, or genital area).
> Moderate or severe pain.

Shingles Complications

Most people do not have any complications. Those that sometimes occur include the following.

Postherpetic Neuralgia (PHN)

This is the most common complication. It is where the nerve pain (neuralgia) of shingles persists after the rash has gone.

Skin Infection

Sometimes the rash becomes infected with germs (bacteria). The surrounding skin then becomes red and tender. If this occurs you may need a course of medicines called antibiotics.

Eye Problems

Shingles of the eye can cause inflammation of the front of the eye. In severe cases it can lead to inflammation of the whole of the eye which may cause loss of vision.

Weakness

Sometimes the nerve affected is a motor nerve (ones which control muscles) and not a usual sensory nerve (ones for touch). This may result in a weakness (palsy) of the muscles that are supplied by the nerve.

Various Other Rare Complications

Examples are infection of the brain by the varicella-zoster virus, or spread of the virus throughout the body. These are very serious but rare. People with a poor immune system (immunosuppression) who develop shingles have a higher than normal risk of developing rare or serious complications. (For example, people with HIV/AIDS, people on chemotherapy, etc.)

Herpes and Shingles Diet

Although shingles is treated through medication, a shingles diet also plays an important role in the prevention and treatment of shingles. A proper diet can help ensure that your immune system is working well. When your immunity is strong, the chances of the Herpes Zoster virus manifesting itself are less. Moreover, this virus affects the nerve endings. Thus, if you are already affected with shingles, it is important to follow a diet for shingles that helps to boost your nervous system.

Antioxidant-rich veggies

Eating vegetables rich in antioxidants can boost your immune system and may minimize inflammation. Cauliflower, spinach, kale, and tomatoes are rich in free-radical binding antioxidants. They also contain more lysine than arginine, an amino acid ratio that's important to suppressing herpes.

Omega-3 fatty acids

Omega 3-chain fatty acids can be used to help your immune system fight chronic inflammatory conditions. Salmon, mackerel, flaxseed, and chia seeds are rich in these fatty acids.

Protein

Consuming a healthy level of protein is vital to fighting off the herpes virus and other pathogens. Keep your diet high in protein and low in saturated fat by eating lots of almonds, eggs, and oats.

Vitamin C

Researchers have demonstrated that vitamin C can efficiently speed the healing of herpes outbreaks. It may also help prolong the time between outbreaks.

Colorful fruits and veggies like bell peppers, oranges, and strawberries are rich in vitamin C.

Mango and papaya fruits also contain the vitamin, without adding a high amount of lysine to your diet.

Zinc

Zinc therapy may reduceTrusted Source the amount of herpes outbreaks you have while giving you a longer time between outbreaks. You can increase the zinc in your diet by eating wheat germ, chick peas, lamb, and pork.

Vitamin B complex

B vitamins can boost your immune response to help your body fight the herpes virus. You can get vitamin B from green beans, eggs, spinach, and broccoli.

Acid

Acidic food may break open cold sores before they're healed. Fruit juice, beer, sodas, and processed foods all tend to be more acidic. Limit these foods and consider water or sparkling seltzer instead.

L-arginine

Avoid foods that contain high levels of arginine whenever you can. Chocolate is particularly rich in this amino acid, which some people claim can trigger herpes symptoms. Satisfy your sweet tooth with a vitamin-dense option like dried mango or apricots, instead.

Added Sugar

Your body converts added sugars to acid. Avoid foods high in added sugar and consider naturally sweet treats, like bananas and oranges, for your desserts.

Processed or preservative heavy

Processed food contains synthetic preservatives that may contribute to oxidative stress. Keeping oxidative stress levels low may help promote healing during outbreaks. Try cutting processed foods like freezer meals, refined grain products, and candies from your diet.

Alcohol

Alcohol breaks down in your body to the equivalent of a sugar. High sugar consumption is linked to white blood cell suppression — which can make outbreaks more likely. If you're going to consume alcohol, do so in moderation, and choose a less acidic beverage, like wine.

Foods To Eat

Let us take a look at some of the foods that should form a part of a diet for shingles:

- Fruits and vegetables provide your body with all the essential micronutrients. Thus, it is important to ensure that you include adequate quantities of fresh fruit and vegetables in your diet. This will help you build and maintain immunity.

- Vitamin B-6 is an important nutrient for those suffering from shingle as it benefits the nerves. Some of the foods that are rich in vitamin B-6 include potatoes, bananas, brewer's yeast and nuts.

- Other foods to eat for a shingles diet include whole grain foods such as brown rice.

- Garlic is a natural source of antioxidants and is a natural antibiotic as well. Try to incorporate garlic into your shingles diet to help heal the blisters faster.

- Lysine is an amino acid that can inhibit the multiplication of Herpes Zoster virus. Some of the good sources of lysine include fish, red meat, dairy products, and beans.

- There are some studies that indicate that consuming seaweed is also an effective way of arresting the spread of the Herpes Zoster virus and thereby preventing shingles.

- Drink lots of water as this will help your body flush out the impurities from your system.

Foods To Avoid

The ratio of the amino acids Arginine to Lysine is the key. Arginine promotes the growth of Herpes and Shingles viruses. Lysine suppresses it. Meats, fats, dairy and vegetables are balanced in Arginine to Lysine.

All Grains are High in Arginine: A grain-free Paleo Diet is the first place to start. It's time to stop bread, flour, pasta, rice, cereal and chips. Stick with Paleo and your immune system and weight will improve.

1). Chocolate

Dark chocolate has many chemical properties, including some that are addictive and brain stimulating (PEA), and others that can support feelings of well-being. BUT, dark chocolate is high in Arginine. The good news is if you're satisfied with a small amount, you're probably OK – unless you're already at the edge of an outbreak.

2). Gelatin and Collagen

OK, don't be alarmed, but gelatin is high in Arginine which is used for many beneficial purposes in the body, including the manufacture of growth hormone. While it may have beneficial properties for many, the Arginine in gelatin and collagen (and bone broth) may not be so great for Herpes sufferers.

elatin may also cause histamine problems. If your allergies, headaches, skin rashes and random "what did I do wrong" issues are not under control, eliminate gelatin for a few weeks and see if things improve.

3). Nuts and Seeds

I am always surprised that sufferers of Herpes or Shingles don't realize that high levels of Arginine in nuts and seeds provoke this virus. I once had a client struggling to get over a persistent Shingles outbreak who quickly improved when she stopped almond butter, bone broth and coconut flour pancakes.

Cashews, pumpkin seeds and macadamia nuts have the best Arginine to Lysine ratio, although it's still not great. Walnuts, sesame seeds, pine nuts, almonds and hazelnuts have the poorest ratio.

This puts a serious damper on almond flour foods and nut and seed snacks. But note....Arginine is not in oils, so almond or macadamia oils are fine as far as Herpes is concerned.

4). Coconut meat, flour and milk

Coconut meat has a good amount of protein (amino acids) and unfortunately a high Arginine to Lysine ratio. Coconut meat is ground up to make coconut flour and canned coconut milk.

Coconut water and coconut oil have no proteins or amino acids and will not affect the herpes virus. They are OK.

Shingles Diet Chart

Here is a sample shingles diet chart that should be followed if you have an outbreak of this disease. Keep in mind that diet is supplementary to medication and should ideally be prescribed by a doctor or nutritionist.

• Breakfast: Try to include eggs in your breakfast as eggs are a rich source of vitamins B1 and B12. Two slices of whole wheat bread and a glass of fresh fruit juice or a bowl of fresh fruit should also be included.

• Lunch: Opt for a high quality protein such as fish. In addition, fresh fruit and vegetables should also be included in good quantities. If you can incorporate seaweed into your diet, it will also be beneficial in a diet for shingles.

• Dinner: Dinner should also be rich in fruit and vegetables. Try to include citrus fruit, carrots, and green leafy vegetables.

• Snacks: Nuts are a good option for snacks in between meals. A glass of milk should also be a part of any diet plan for shingles.

Shingles Health Tips

In addition to taking the right medication and consuming a proper diet for shingles, it is also important to avoid stress. Excess of stress can also suppress the immune system and allow the dormant Herpes Zoster virus to initiate an attack of shingles. It is also a good idea to identify situations that trigger stress attacks and avoid or minimize them. Counseling can also help you deal with stress. Regular exercise and sleep also help to alleviate stress.

Conclusion

These two diseases are different right from their causative agents, and up to their signs and symptoms, all the way to their methods of treatment.

The factual and scientific differences that exist serve to render shingles and herpes as being different diseases, contrary to what some may think. Shingles and herpes, also referred to as herpes zoster and herpes simplex respectively, however share the same family of viruses, herein the herpes virus. This is where there similarity begins and ends, and when it comes to the medical basics of both diseases as above-mentioned and detailed, one's eyes will truly be opened to see that indeed, they are distinct. Shingles and herpes are different, and that is a proven and tested fact.

Based on the fact that these two diseases are in fact viral and can not be ridden from a patient's body in totality once acquired, we offer advice by asserting the old adage that indeed prevention is better than cure, and the best treatment for the aforementioned diseases would be to refrain from unprotected sexual encounters.